AUTHOR'S BIOGRAPHY: Professor Edward Glassman, Ph.D.

Taught NUTRITION for 12 years as a Professor (now retired) in the Biochemistry and Nutrition Department of the Medical School in the University of North Carolina in Chapel Hill, NC (1960-1989). He published over 100 research articles on biochemistry, genetics; neuroscience; alcohol; teaching; and creativity.

Born March 18, 1929 in NYC and graduated from Stuyvesant High School in 1946, Professor Edward Glassman received his Ph.D. in 1955 from the Biology Department in The Johns Hopkins University, Baltimore, Maryland.

He was a Guggenheim Fellow and Visiting Professor at Stanford University, Palo Alto, California (1968-1969; Visiting Professor, University of California; Irvine, California (1978); Visiting Fellow; Center For Creative Leadership; Greensboro, North Carolina (1982); and Visiting Scientist, Stanford Research Center (SRI) Menlo Park, Calif (1986).

He served on the Editorial Board of "Neurochemical Research" (1975-1978); "Behavioral Biology" (1971-1976); "Pharmacology, Biochemistry, and Behavior" (1973-1988); "Behavior Genetics" (1970-1971).

He served as a Postdoctoral Fellow of the American Cancer Society in the Biology Department of California Institute of Technology, Pasadena, California (1955-1957); and a Postdoctoral Fellow of the National Institutes of Health in the Genetics Department at the Universities of Edinburgh and Zurich (1958-1959).

From 1992 to 1997, he was a Columnist for newspapers in Chapel Hill, Raleigh; and Moore County, North Carolina.

SENIOR CITIZEN'S GUIDE TO LOSING WEIGHT:

You Really Do Want To Lose Weight, Don't You?

By Edward Glassman, Ph.D.

--A Personal View--

SENIOR CITIZENS OFTEN FIND IT DIFFICULT TO LOSE WEIGHT

Lets face it, most people find it hard to lose weight, and senior citizens even more so, mainly because they become less active, do not realize that their body requires less calories than when they were younger and therefore requires less food, and they sometimes forget that longevity and mental agility depends partly on being thin.

This book is dedicated to all who wish to lose weight, and keep it off, and want to do it with a purpose.

Ed Glassman, March 18, 2014

CreateSpace

https://www.createspace.com/4656510

Before you make significant changes to your nutrition or exercise, please consult your Doctor and other health professionals for your safety.

Although we have insured the accuracy of the information in this book, we assume no responsibility for errors, inaccuracies, omissions, or other inconsistencies here.

©2014 by Edward Glassman

Create Space
https://www.createspace.com/4656510

ISBN-13: 978-1495455193

All rights reserved.

PLEASE DO NOT DUPLICATE ANY MATERIAL IN THIS BOOK
WITHOUT WRITTEN PERMISSION.

No part of this book may be reproduced in any form or by any electronic or mechanical means, including information storage or retrieval systems without permission in written form from the author; except by a reviewer, who may quote brief passages in a review; and except for individual use if credit is given to Edward Glassman and to this book. Inclusion of items in publications for sale or profit is permitted only with prior written permission.

TABLE OF CONTENTS

- Nothing Feels As Good As Being Thin Feels
- Your Lifestyle Makeover Will Require Tough Love From You
- A Current Source of Easy-To-Understand Nutrition Information
- Warning (again)...
- Finally...
- It's A Nutrient Numbers Nightmare
- You Need 'Tough Love' & Discipline To Lose Weight And Keep It Off
- And Now...

III.
EATING RIGHT: Lose Weight & Feel Fit   23

- Eating Right Is A Nutrition Numbers Nightmare
- People Eat All Kinds Of Food
- Eat For Health, Fitness & Vitality

· ACTIVITY TABLE #1:

    List All The Foods You Ate Yesterday.

- Nutrients In the Food You Eat
- Nutrition Facts Label
- Examples of 'Nutrition Facts' Labels

· ACTIVITY TABLE #2

Calculate The Nutrient Content Of The Foods You Listed In Table 1.

· ACTIVITY TABLE #3:

Calculate The Total Amount Of Each Nutrient You Listed in Table 2.

How Much of Each Nutrient Below Do You Require Each Day (the Daily Value-DV)?

Calories

% Calories From Fat

Saturated Fat

Polyunsaturated

Fat

Monosaturated Fat

Cholesterol

Sodium

Potassium

Carbohydrates

Fiber

Sugars

Protein

Vitamins, Minerals, &

Antioxidants

Water

Eating Right For Longevity

Do You Know How Much Of These Nutrients You Require Each Day?

- ACTIVITY TABLE #4:

    List Your Daily Required Amounts of the Nutrients Listed In the 'Nutrition Facts' Label.

- ACTIVITY TABLE #5:

    Determine the adequacy of the nutrients in the food you listed in Table 4 by comparing it with Table 1.

- ACTIVITY TABLE #6:

    Devise A Daily Menu Plan That Provides You With The Nutrients You Require.

- Give Yourself 'Tough Love'
- You Won't Lose Much Weight Working Out
- Warm Up To Prevent Injury
- Cool Down & Stretch When Finished
- Dehydration
- More Awesome Books
- A Schedule To Start Eating And Working Out Right.

I. INTRODUCTION

NUTRITION IS A NUMBERS NIGHTMARE

While fine cooking belongs to the arts, and inspired eating belongs to the gourmets, good nutrition depends on numbers:

- How much of each essential nutrient do you require each day?
- How much of each essential nutrient do you take in each day?
- How much more, or less, of each essential nutrient do you need to take in?

This book will take you painlessly through these numbers so you may make better choices about what you eat, and moreover, about changes you may want to carry over to your current lifestyle.

MY PERSONAL VIEW OF MY NUTRITION

This book presents my personal view and practice of my personal nutrition, my attempt to eat right while I control my weight, and my personal experiences during numerous sessions working out to tone my muscles and strengthen my body. My purpose in writing about it, you ask? I wrote it to summarize my crazy (like a fox) diet for my daughters and my grandchildren so they can consider it and decide for themselves what they choose. I hope they will learn at least one life-altering lesson, although I have humble thoughts about this prospect.

I also wrote it so you may also consider it and decide for yourself whether you can benefit from it. Personally, I believe the information I included in this book will help you lose, and then maintain, your weight in a healthy way.

'TRY IT AND CHOOSE FOR YOURSELF'

'Try it and choose for yourself' permeates this book because the science of human nutrition suffers from a number of disadvantages.

First, every person's biochemistry varies from time to time with age, food intake, gender, activity, and from person to person, so setting rigid standards for nutrition, or for anything else related to biochemistry, seems tenuous, at best.

Second, nutritional experiments on humans are very difficult and expensive to carry out with adequate controls and statistical significance, and take a long time.

Third, the media and the lay public desires hard, concrete, never-changing facts so they know exactly what to eat, forever. When so-called facts change with new data, the media and the public rebel, and the science suffers.

Instead of relying on changeable scientific data, I experimented with my food while I stayed within the limits of good sense and good science. I had the knowledge to do this because I taught Nutrition for 12 years in the Department of Biochemistry and Nutrition at the University of North Carolina at Chapel Hill, where I retired as Professor Emeritus in 1989. I pass my current food habits on in this book.

Stay flexible. Many of us stick to the food habits we learned as a child or as a newlywed, and resist change. If this works for you, fine. If your eating habits do not work for you, and you want to lose weight & keep it off, then this book presents an opportunity to try other approaches and choose for yourself.

FITNESS, VITALITY, & TOUGH LOVE

Fitness & vitality mean different things to different people. To me, they mean the ability to...
- walk 3 miles on the treadmill
- have adequate muscle strength
- work out 3 days a week
- respond well to stress
- enjoy the daily experience of eating right
- avoid colds and other minor illnesses
- control my weight and look trim
- have the stamina and endurance to enjoy life
- feel good with a high sense of well being
- maintain a cool head

To attain these abilities, consider a lifestyle makeover, a change in lifestyle that involves new eating habits, working out regularly; new relationship skills, meditation, yoga, more fun, etc. Not to worry. This book will guide you through learning to eat and work out right; the rest you can find elsewhere (see, for example: "Vitality Challenge" by Art Ulene; Published by Black Diamond Associates; 2002).

To attain a lifestyle makeover, you may have to apply "tough love" and determination to confront yourself and others when you or they interfere with your goals. "Tough love" can work if you commit yourself to attaining fitness and vitality. Go ahead, COMMIT...

ACKNOWLEDGMENTS

I want to thank the outstanding Vicki Bradley, my four marvelous daughters, and my wonderful grandchildren for their totally effective support and encouragement.

I also want to express my gratitude and admiration to Randy Ballard, my trainer for the past 8 years, for his effectiveness in helping me become more fit and more vital than I thought possible. His patience and "tough love" contributed wonderfully to my relatively pain-free workouts with him, which now number more than 800, so many opportunities to develop.

Thanks also to Dave Jolliffe, my once and future training partner and always an intelligent companion, for his knowledge and generous sharing of all things worthy. To him & his wife Joan, and to Vicki, many gratitudes for a splendid job editing this book.

THE ORGANIZATION OF THIS BOOK

You will discover repetition in this book 'over and over again.' I did this so the message sinks in, and you 'totally get it.'

I organized the book by simplifying the science, so it hardly interferes, and boxing the numbers so they appear less formidable. First, I present my Personal Simpler Approach to eat right so I lose weight and keep it off.

Then I present details of 'Eating Right' and 'Working Out.' These topics go together like a hand in a glove. You must not do one without the other. Promise you won't.

At the end, I present the **APPENDICES**, which contain many interesting ideas. For example, the Appendices deal with diverse topics, like: I. Eating for alertness, II. Foods that fill you up, III. Classroom materials I handed out in 1984, and V. How to navigate the Nutrition Facts labels; all good stuff.

Throughout the 'Eating Right' section of this book, I present **ACTIVITY TABLES** to trigger your thoughts concerning the nutrients in the food you eat. These tables derive from a course I taught on nutrition. Each Table will help you understand your nutritional needs, and how to manage them. I boxed them to help you organize the information you put in them.

Furthermore, these Activity Tables may be used to help members of your family and friends to analyze their nutrition, and whether they eat right, taking in all the recommended daily amounts of nutrients.

In addition, another topic slithers through this book: 'Tough Love.' It means disciplining yourself to do things even though they make you feel uncomfortable, like a 'Lifestyle Makeover' (another topic), a very difficult thing to accomplish and which requires all the support you can get.

Also, look for references to ...

But enough of this. Let us move on to the heart of the matter, 'My Personal Approach to Weight Loss,' 'Eating Right' ... And then, 'Working Out.'

II. MY SIMPLER APPROACH TO EATING RIGHT

LOSING WEIGHT & KEEPING IT OFF IS A NUTRITION NUMBERS GAME

To lose weight in a healthy manner requires knowing a way to reduce the number of calories you need without reducing the intake of essential nutrients. The numbers include the following:

• What is the minimum number of calories you may safely eat daily to lose weight?

• How can you reduce the number of calories you eat each day and still be sure you get the required amount of each essential nutrient?

A SIMPLIFIED 'CRAZY (like a fox) DIET PLAN'

I have been experimenting with my food intake for more than 35 years and I know that constant calculation involves tedious hours of frustration. In the end, I developed a simpler diet that suits me well. Modify it to suit yourself. Perhaps our goals match.

• To lose weight & keep it off

• Know I have taken in the recommended daily amounts of my required nutrients

• Eat good-mood foods (high protein)

• Eat enough protein to maintain my muscle mass

- Not feel stuffed
- Tastes good
- Enjoyable

SUMMARY: My simpler approach to losing weight & keeping it off involves consuming my daily required nutrients in food containing a total of about 720 calories. This allows me to supplement my intake with small snacks that supply the additional calories I need to accomplish my goals, either to lose weight, gain weight, or maintain my weight. By weighing myself every other day at the same time of day, I obtain feedback on how well I succeed in moving towards my weight goals.

This book provides the nutritional numbers and a detailed analysis of my approach, so you can modify it to fit your goals.

BREAKFAST

I like the following breakfast because it achieves my goals:
- high protein to elevate my mood
- low fat & low bulk so I don't feel stuffed
- high fiber
- good taste
- enough calories to start the day

To achieve these goals during breakfast, I stir together and consume:

- one-quarter cup of Fiber One cereal
- one ounce of 100% whey Protein Powder (chocolate)
- one cup of Skim Milk

The Nutrition Facts label for one cup of **Skim Milk** ...

Calories:	80
Calories from fat:	0
Total fat:	0 g (grams)
Saturated fat:	0 g
Trans fat:	0 g
Polyunsaturated fat:	0 g
Monosaturated fat:	0 g
Cholesterol:	<5 mg
Sodium:	125 mg
Potassium:	N/A
Total carbohydrate:	12 g
Dietary fiber:	0 g
Soluble fiber:	N/A
Sugars:	12 g
Other carbohydrates:	N/A
Protein:	8 g
Vitamins % Daily Values:	N/A
Minerals % Daily Values:	N/A

To find out more about the Nutrition Facts labels, see pages 25 & 53.

The Nutrition Facts label for one-quarter cup of **Fiber One cereal** looks like this ...

Calories:	60 cal
Calories from fat:	10 ca
Total fat:	1 g (grams)
Saturated fat:	<0 g
Trans fat:	<0 g
Polyunsaturated fat:	<0 g
Monosaturated fat:	<0 g
Cholesterol:	0 mg
Sodium:	105 mg
Potassium:	180 mg
Total carbohydrate:	25 g
Dietary fiber:	14 g
Soluble fiber:	1 g
Sugars:	0 g
Other carbohydrates:	11 g
Protein:	2 g
Vitamins % Daily Values:	N/A
Minerals % Daily Values:	N/A

The Nutrition Facts label for 1 ounce of **100% whey Protein Powder** looks like this...

Calories:	100 cal
Calories from fat:	5
Total fat:	<1 g (grams)
Saturated fat:	<0.5 g
Trans fat:	<1 g
Polyunsaturated fat:	N/A
Monosaturated fat:	N/A
Cholesterol:	10 mg
Sodium:	75 mg
Potassium:	N/A
Calcium:	50 mg
Total carbohydrate:	8 g
Dietary fiber:	<1 g
Soluble fiber:	N/A
Sugars:	6 g
Other carbohydrates:	N/A
Protein:	16 g
Vitamins % Daily Values:	N/A
Minerals % Daily Values:	N/A

I ALSO TAKE IN DURING AND AFTER breakfast ...
- 1 tablet containing all required vitamins and minerals.

- 1 tablet: selenium   200 mcg

- 1 tablet: vitamin C   250 mg

- 1 tablet: B-50 complex   50 mg each of 11 B-vitamins.

- 1 tablet: Omega-3 fish oil   1000 mg

- 1 tablet vitamin D   400 IU, every other day.

- water   2 glasses

The TOTAL amount of nutrients in **MY BREAKFAST**...

Calories:	240 cal
Calories from fat:	15 cal
Total fat:	<2 g
Saturated fat:	>0 g N/A
Trans fat:	>0 g N/A
Polyunsaturated fat:	>0 g N/A
Monosaturated fat:	>0 g N/A
Cholesterol:	10 mg
Sodium:	305 mg
Potassium;	<180 mg N/A
Total carbohydrate:	45 g
Dietary fiber:	15 g
Soluble fiber:	>1 g N/A
Sugars:	>18 g
Other carbohydrates:	>11 g N/A
Protein:	26 g
Vitamins % Daily Values:	all
Minerals % Daily Values:	all

LUNCH & DINNER:

I repeat breakfast at lunch and dinner, omitting the tablets. Total nutrients in my lunch and dinner equals the same as breakfast, except I do NOT take in any tablets of vitamins and minerals, or antioxidant.

MINIMUM AMOUNT OF NUTRIENTS I EAT EACH DAY

Calories:	720
Calories from fat:	45
Total fat:	4 g (grams)
Saturated fat:	<0 g
Trans fat:	<0 g
Polyunsaturated fat:	<0 g
Monosaturated fat:	<0 g
Cholesterol:	30 mg
Sodium:	915 mg
Potassium:	N/A
Total carbohydrate:	136 g
Dietary fiber:	45 g
Soluble fiber:	N/A
Sugars:	54 g
Other carbohydrates:	N/A
Protein:	78 g
Vitamins % Daily Values:	all
Minerals % Daily Values:	all
Antioxidants:	some
Water:	4 to 6 glasses.

Please note that I do not vary this minimum daily food intake described above. Its main deficiency comprises the 720 calories, and I want to exceed 2.5 times that amount.

WHERE DO I OBTAIN MORE CALORIES?

I obtain additional calories by eating small portions of the following snacks throughout the day: pasta; bread, cheese; fruit; vegetables; salad; tomato and cucumber salad; tofu; applesauce; raisins; grains (rice, barley, kasha; quinoa, couscous); fish; chicken; turkey; almonds; prunes; potato; peanut butter; a rare bit of chocolate, etc.

I eat small snacks, not full meals. Otherwise, they would undermine my goal of losing weight & keeping it off. But how do I determine how much of the snacks I will eat? I weigh myself every other day, at the same time of day. If my weight trends upwards, I eat less; if it trends downward, I eat more. In other words, I use the feedback of my weight to tell me how much snack food I should eat each day.

After breakfast, on days that I work out, I need extra calories, so I eat these foods:
One 'Pure Protein' bar; plus one ounce of almonds; plus one slice of bread. These three foods provide the extra calories that I need while I work out.

The Nutrition Facts label for my '**Pure Protein' bar** looks like this...

200	calories
45	calories from fat
5 g	total fat
3 g	saturated fat
0 g	trans fat
10 mg	cholesterol
85 mg	sodium
20 mg	potassium
18 g	carbohydrate
0 g	fiber
3 g	sugars
7 g	sugar alcohol
20 g	protein
	assorted vitamins and minerals

This 'Pure Protein' bar has a low ratio of calories to grams of protein: 200 calories to 20 grams of protein, or 10 to 1. Some so-called high protein bars have ratios of calories to grams of protein as high as 25 to 1, too many calories per gram of protein.

The Nutrition Facts label for **one ounce of nuts (22-23 almonds)** looks like this...

169	calories
125	calories from fat
15g	fat
1 g	saturated fat
0 g	trans fat
0 g	cholesterol
0 mg	sodium
5 g	total carbohydrate
3 g	fiber
1 g	sugar
6 g	protein

The Nutrition Facts label for **one medium slice of bread ...**

80-100*	calories,
5-10*	calories from fat,
1 g	total fat,
0 g	saturated or trans fat,
0 g	cholesterol,
120-180 mg*	sodium,
12-16 g*	carbohydrate,
1-2 g	fiber,
1-2 g	sugars,
1-4 g*	protein

*depends on the bread

These three foods (protein bar, almonds, and bread) provide the extra calories that I need while I work out,

What do I do in a restaurant where I lack control over ingredients and size of the portions? I order a high protein appetizer, usually small and delicious, and a glass of water with some bread. I told you discipline would factor heavily in eating right.

What do I eat on a road trip? I refuse to eat fast food. Instead, whenever hunger strikes, I eat 8 to 10 almonds or half a 'Pure Protein' bar described above.

Nine almonds contain, as shown on the Nutrition Facts label...

52	calories
38	calories from polyunsaturated fat
0	trans fat
5 g	fat
0 g	cholesterol
3 mg	sodium,
2 g	carbohydrate
1 g	fiber
0 g	sugars
2 g	protein

While I experimented with my food intake over the years, I worked out in fitness centers two to four afternoons a week for about 35 years. Also, for the past 8 years, I trained with a personal trainer two afternoons a week and worked out an extra afternoon per week on my own. I still do, and in addition, I do cardiovascular training on the treadmill for about an hour each time I go the fitness center.

MY RESULTS

The result of my working out and eating diets similar to the one I described in this book pleases and amazes me. Although 85 years old, I have good health, and rarely miss a workout because of illness (only about four to five times in the past eight years). I almost never get a cold, and my annual physical checkup reports come back negative. I recently lost 35 pounds and now weigh 148 pounds; my body looks slim. I have toned muscles, and a sense of well being; I feel good and fit.

TRY THIS AND DECIDE FOR YOURSELF

Too good to be true? Will this work for you? Try it and choose for yourself.

Start by consulting your doctor. Get her or his okay. Start taking a complete vitamins & minerals tablet once a day. Arrange to work out with a personal trainer, either alone or with a group of friends to share fees. Start to weigh yourself at the same time every other day. Reduce food intake so you lose about 1 to 2 pounds a week, never more than that, or you will lose muscle tissue (except at the beginning when you will lose water).

Reduce food portion size by half; cut out desserts; cut down on fatty foods eventually eliminating them entirely; leave out salt. And reduce your intake of sugar, and bread & butter.

Do not diet unless you also work out; otherwise, you may lose muscle mass. And make sure you take in enough protein and carbohydrate so you will not lose tissue mass, your body's effort to preserve your brain and nervous system.

Eventually develop a menu plan that provides you with the nutrients you require each day with a minimum of calories so you can control your weight, as I did. Arrange your food intake so you can repeat it every day, and supplement it with one vitamin and mineral tablet and selected delicious and balanced snacks each day. In this way, you can lose weight & keep it off.

STOP FOOD TEMPTATION

Food temptation comes in three tasty flavors: sugar, salt, and fat, all potentially harmful to your goal to eat right. These tasty flavors predominate in fast food, canned goods, restaurants, and your kitchen.

Do not tempt yourself. Remove all fattening foods from your home: junk food, candy, desserts, cookies, cake, chocolate, fatty foods, sugar, (and salt), etc.

SOME SIMPLE BIOCHEMISTRY ABOUT WEIGHT REDUCTION

Dieting to lose weight puts a stress on your body's biochemistry. As you reduce your intake of calories, your body seeks to protect the brain's structural integrity from breaking down.

Your body does this by breaking down other tissues to supply the brain with glucose for chemical energy, and with amino acids for protein. You seek to lose fat, not protein. Unfortunately, the body does not know this and breaks down tissue protein too.

The brain can only use glucose as its major energy source. Unfortunately, humans cannot convert fat into glucose (or protein), so your body breaks down tissues like heart, lung, liver, kidney, glands, and muscle, to get glucose and amino acids for the nervous system.

Thus, you run the risk of reducing your muscles and other tissues made of protein to provide amino acids and glucose to your brain.

When dieting to lose weight, you must, therefore, eat adequate amounts of protein to minimize the breakdown of your muscles and other tissues, and enough glucose (carbohydrate) to supply energy to the brain.

Eating right by following my personal food intake plan helps in this regard by supplying a minimum of 75 g of protein and 136 g of carbohydrate per day.

In addition, working out 3 times a week helps tone and build muscles, so you minimize muscle loss while you lose weight.

COPY THE ESSENCE OF MY APPROACH

Develop you own simplified plan to eat right while losing weight. Devise a one day menu in which you take in the required amounts of nutrients with a minimum of calories, as I did. Include what you will eat in restaurants, on road trips, at dinner parties and holiday feasts. Plan to work out regularly. Start a lifestyle makeover.

NOTHING FEELS AS GOOD AS BEING THIN FEELS

How motivated are you to start a lifestyle makeover? Choose which you prefer:

- Feeling good because you just had a great meal...or feeling good because you see yourself as thin & fit? Over the long haul you cannot have both.
- Feeling bad because you gave up overeating at holiday feasts and dinner parties...or feeling bad because you are overweight, with diabetes, heart disease, stroke, high blood pressure, or any of the ailments associated with being overweight? Which?
- Felling great because you finally lost one pound...or feeling great because you finally possess a way to lose weight & keep it off, and to control your weight so it doesn't control you.

The consequences of poor eating habits sticks to us all our lives. Commit now to dramatically improve your poor eating habits for your own sake.

YOUR LIFESTYLE MAKEOVER WILL REQUIRE 'TOUGH LOVE' FROM YOU

Most of us find it hard to change even a little. But...a lifestyle makeover? Nearly impossible. Still, worth investigating? A lifestyle makeover requires the development of new skill sets:

- eating right daily;
- working out regularly (no more excuses);
- relaxing meditation skills;
- better relationship skills;
- more positive approaches to life;
- seeking more fun;
- Avoiding harmful substances, like alcohol and other drugs
- etc.

This book discusses eating right and working out; the rest you can learn elsewhere. Never stop changing. You may find it enjoyable, even fun. And your self esteem may go through the roof as you add new skill sets to your repertoire of life.

A CURRENT, ONGOING SOURCE OF EASY-TO-UNDERSTAND, SUPERIOR, NUTRITION INFORMATION

Subscribe to: "Nutrition Action Healthletter," published by The Center for Science in the Public Interest, Suite 300, 1875 Connecticut Avenue, N.W. Washington, DC 20009; $24 / year. Easily the best ongoing source of nutrition information for the layperson (and myself) that I know. A necessity.

ALSO: check out nutritiondata.com on your computer, a web site that provides a huge amount of food information, including Nutrition Facts for many thousands of foods. Don't leave home without it.

ALSO: check out 'Nutritive Value Of Food' published by the US Department of Agriculture. For sale by the Superintendent of Documents, U.S. Government Printing Office. Internet: bookstore.gpo.gov/   Phone: toll free (866) 512-1800.

WARNING... Do not diet to lose weight...
- unless you consult your doctor first.
- unless you also work out, so you maintain your muscle mass.
- unless you eat enough extra protein to ensure your body will not break down your tissues, such as your heart, kidneys, glands, liver, muscles, etc.

FINALLY...vow to change your lifestyle:
• start a lifestyle makeover
• eat right at every meal
• work out often
• control your weight
• meditate daily
• lower stress
• have more fun
The outcome will amaze and delight you.

IT'S A NUTRIENT NUMBERS NIGHTMARE

Please choose... Well, maybe not choose yet, just pay attention...

This book presents a different way to look at nutrition. Most nutritionists, including my younger self, view nutrition advice in terms of individual foods or categories of foods, such as meats, vegetables, desserts, grains, bread, beans, cereals, fruits, juices, diary, milk, and often present nutritional advice in the simplified form of balanced food groups.

On the other hand, you could choose to skip that layer of perception and focus directly on the nutrients that you require each day, the Daily Values (DV). These represent the required amounts of each nutrient you need every day. Focusing on the nutrients, rather than on foods and food groups, enables you to construct a meal plan that simplifies planning and calculating, and enables you to lose weight & keep it off.

What do I have against the food category approach, that nightmare approach? The endless and tedious calculations and planning take too much time, produce too much frustration, and at the end of the day, I still do not know if I obtained the required amount of nutrients.

Experts have complained about my focus on nutrients. First, they think I would be bored eating the same foods three times a day, every day. Second, they fear I do not eat a balanced diet. Third, they have doubts about the discipline and focus my approach requires. These observations miss the point, actually miss many points.

They fail to see that my approach enables me to take in all the nutrients I require each day with an intake containing only 720 calories, and that each day, I consume about 1,000 calories of delicious snacks, quite balanced, and not boring at all. In fact, very comforting.

Furthermore, I feel good. Nothing feels as good as being thin feels. This motivation fuels its own discipline.

In addition, some people claim that undiscovered nutrients exist and that I risk a harmful deficiency with the way I eat. I guess they think a balanced diet would prevent me from developing a deficiency in the unknown nutrients.

The thought that unknown nutrients exist constitutes wishful thinking. Surely 100 years of nutrition research brought forth the major nutrients. And if anyone should show deficiency symptoms, it certainly would be me. Instead, no deficiency.

One person actually said I would have even greater health if I ate more sensibly. Well, I do eat sensibly and would love greater health, Still, how much health can I achieve at 84 years of age.

YOU NEED 'TOUGH LOVE' & DISCIPLINE TO LOSE WEIGHT AND KEEP IT OFF

Now choose for yourself.
• You do want to lose weight, and then keep the pounds from returning, don't you?
• And you do want to feel fit, full of vitality, don't you?
• And you do want to simplify the eating process and have confidence that, at the end of the day, you take in the required amounts of the nutrients you need, don't you?
• And you do want to experience comfort with your diet, the comfort diet, don't you?
If so, what holds you back?

AND NOW...
Please move on to learn more about losing weight and keeping it off by eating right.

III. EATING RIGHT: Lose Weight & Feel Fit

EATING RIGHT IS A NUTRITION NUMBERS NIGHTMARE

By 'eating right' I refer to eating the kind and amount of foods that maximizes your health, well being, longevity, and quality of life. Given the increase in obesity and diabetes, to name a few instances, many people do not appear to eat right.

Eating right is in the numbers.

• How much of each essential nutrient do you require?

• How much of each essential nutrient do you take in each day?

• How much more, or less, of each essential nutrient do you need each day?

In this section of this book you find out how these numbers affect you.

PEOPLE EAT ALL KINDS OF FOODS

People all over the world eat such a variety of foods that it becomes difficult to chart a universal norm. Surely, a Swede eats different food than an African native; a native living in the rain forest eats differently from a Bedouin in the desert; before 1900, an Inuit (Eskimo) rarely ate fruits and vegetables during the winter, subsisting mainly on fish and fat (blubber), while an inhabitant of the United States eats richly.

And a Native-American eats quite different foods from a native Indian, who eats differently from a native of Indonesia, Vietnam, China or Japan.

Even within the United States, food habits vary in different regions, although widespread similar supermarkets trim the degree of difference: people who live along the coast eat differently from those in the heartland; Northerners eat differently from Southerners; vegetarians do not eat meat, while others crave it. Some people eat according to religious tenets, while others eat 'fast food.' Some eat sparingly to lose or maintain weight, while others gorge themselves.

For most people, what they eat usually represents habits they learned as a child, and which they only changed slightly as they age. This book will help you evaluate what you eat, and how to eat more effectively.

EAT FOR HEALTH, FITNESS, & VITALITY

Who wins the prize for eating right? People must meet one major criterion to judge whether they eat right: they reproduce, which is nature's prime requirement for eating right. However, another human criterion exists for eating right: quality of life. You define this best for yourself, but almost everyone would include health, fitness, and vitality as one goal of eating right. And many people would include looking trim, feeling good (a sense of well being), and a control over body weight.

If these goals define your wishes, you have come to the right place. When you finish reading this book, and doing what it asks in the Activity Tables, you will have a good idea of how to achieve these goals. In addition, you will understand what you have to give up to attain them (probably holiday feasts, food binges, alcohol, some fun, etc.). Now please fill out Activity Table 1.

ACTIVITY TABLE #1.

List All The Foods You Ate Yesterday (or any recent day).

Breakfast:

Lunch:

Dinner:

Snacks:

Water:

Did you forget anything? Drinks? Candy? Late night snack?

Comments:

NUTRIENTS IN THE FOOD YOU EAT

You can discover the nutrients in the food you eat in the 'Nutrition Facts' printed on every food can or package. Also see the 'Nutrient Tables' published in books or available in computer programs. One excellent, convenient, internet source lists the nutrients in the food you eat: **nutritiondata.com**. This handy website provides you with 'Nutrients Facts' on most foods. Bookmark & and save it. See also: Nutrition Facts Desk Reference" by Art Ulene; Avery Publishing, 785 pages (1995).

SAMPLE of a Nutrition Facts Label

*Taken from the USDA

Nutrition Facts

Serving Size 1 cup (228g)
Servings Per Container 2

Amount Per Serving

Calories 260   Calories from fat 120

% Daily Value*

Total Fat 13g	**20%**
Saturated Fat 5g	**25%**
Cholesterol 30mg	**10%**
Sodium 660mg	**28%**
Total Carbohydrate 31g	**10%**
Dietary Fiber 0g	**0%**
Sugars 5g	
Protein 5g	

Vitamin A 4%   ●   Vitamin C 2%

Calcium 15%   ●   Iron 4%

* Percent Daily Values are based on a 2,000
calorie diet. Your daily value may be higher
or lower depending on your calorie needs:

		Calories:	2,000	2,500
Total Fat	Less than		65g	80g
Sat Fat	Less than		20g	25g
Cholesterol	Less than		300mg	300mg
Sodium	Less than		2,400mg	2,400mg
Total Carbohydrate			300g	375g
Dietary Fiber			25g	30g

Calories per gram:
Fat 9 * Carbohydrate 4 * Protein 4

'NUTRITION FACTS' LABEL (see also Appendix IV):

The Nutrition Facts printed on almost all food sold in the USA supply the following information about the nutrients in your food:

Serving size and servings per container:

Calories:	cal (calories)
Calories from fat:	cal
Total fat:	g (grams)
Saturated fat:	g
Trans fat:	g
Polyunsaturated fat:	g
Monosaturated fat:	g
Cholesterol:	mg (milligrams)
Sodium:	mg
Potassium:	mg
Total carbohydrate:	g
Dietary fiber:	g
Soluble fiber:	g
Sugars:	g
Other carbohydrates:	g
Protein:	g
Vitamins	% Daily Values (% DV)
Minerals:	% Daily Values (% DV)

INGREDIENTS: (the items with the largest amounts by weight listed first):

ACTIVITY TABLE #2.

Calculate The Nutrients In Each Food You Listed In Activity Table 1.

Breakfast:

Lunch:

Dinner:

Snacks:

Include drinks, candy and water:

Comments:

ACTIVITY TABLE #3.

Calculate The Total Amount of Each Nutrient In The Food You Listed In Activity Table 2.

Calories:	cal
Calories from fat:	cal
Total fat:	g (grams)
Saturated fat:	g
Trans fat:	g
Polyunsaturated fat:	g
Monosaturated fat:	g
Cholesterol:	mg
Sodium:	mg
Potassium:	mg
Total carbohydrate:	g
Dietary fiber:	g
Soluble fiber:	g
Sugars:	g
Other carbohydrates:	g
Protein:	g
Vitamins:	% Daily Values (% DV)
Minerals:	% Daily Values (% DV)
Water:	glasses each day

Comments:

HOW MUCH OF EACH NUTRIENT DO YOU NEED EACH DAY?

Listing the essential nutrients in your food provides useful information, but you need to know more to judge the adequacy of your food. You also need to know how much of each nutrient you require each day. The USDA refers to this number as the Daily Value (DV), and the percent of this number that exists in each food represents the % Daily Value (% DV).

The exact amount that we need of each nutrient varies according to age, sex, height, weight, activity (sedentary, active, athletic), weather, health, etc. So, any attempt at exactness merely provides a good guess.

Nonetheless, you can make use of good sense and good science to judge the adequacy of what you eat as you endeavor to lose and then control your weight, enhancing your fitness and well-being.

The following discusses the required daily amounts of most of the nutrients found on the 'Nutrition Facts' label:

CALORIES

All nutrients, except minerals, can turn into chemical calories to fuel your body's chemistry, unless your body excretes them. The number of calories required by your body varies with size, weight, sex, age, activity, nutritional goals, etc.

You can monitor the effectiveness of the calories you eat by weighing yourself at the same time every other day, and watching the trend of your body's weight.

Thus, if you want to lose weight, eat less so your weight trends downward. If you want to gain weight, eat more so your weight trends upward. Thus, you can control your weight (up, down, steady) using "tough love" based on the trend of your weight.

You can also affect the trend of your weight by directly controlling the number of calories you eat. Look up the foods you eat in the Nutrient Tables described above. A tedious method, it does not equal the feedback power or the convenience of the weight trend method.

You can roughly guess how many calories you need each day to keep your weight steady by the following method: Multiply your weight in pounds x 12 if you have a sedentary lifestyle; multiply x 15 if you carry out moderate activities; and x 18 if you perform athletics daily. The number you calculate provides you with a rough estimate of the calories you need per day. This quick calculation may provide you with an estimate that helps you better interpret the feedback from your every-other-day weighing.

As we age over 30 years old, our body's metabolism requires less and less calories, about 1% less per year. This may not seem like much, but it means 10% less per decade, and 30% less between 20 and 50 years old. This explains why people gain weight, sometimes massively, as they age. So, lower the number of calories you consume daily as you age if you want to prevent excessive weight gain.

Seasonal athletes put on weight because they require less calories during the off-season, and after they retire. During the season, their caloric needs are high because they are so active, and they need to eat a lot to maintain their weight. During the off season, and after retirement, they are less active. Unless they cut their caloric intake, they will put on weight.

% CALORIES FROM FAT

To aid in judging a food, the government mandates that the Nutrition Facts on each food's package include the percentage of calories from fat, listed as saturated fat, trans fat, polyunsaturated fat, and monosaturated fat. I tend not to eat foods that have a high percentage of calories from fat, except for nuts that have a high percentage of polyunsaturated fat.

TOTAL FAT

Nutritionist struggle over our need to eat fat. Please let them fight it out. I reduce my intake of fat as low as I can. I have never heard of a fat deficiency occurring in the USA (or anywhere else). I take a capsule containing Omega-3 fish oil daily, because of reports that it lowers the risk of heart attacks and stroke.

SATURATED FAT

Fat makes for complex chemistry. Please believe me that we do not want to discuss its structure here. Take it as true that you want to reduce your intake of saturated fat. I avoid it. It inhabits mammalian meat and coconuts. Medical scientists think high amounts of saturated fat lead to higher levels of cholesterol in blood, and consequent heart attacks and strokes.

POLYUNSATURATED FAT

This fat inhabits plants (and nuts). Medical scientists believe this fat lowers cholesterol in blood, and reduces consequent heart disease and stroke.

MONOSATURATED FAT

Nutritionists believe that monosaturated fat, found in olives and olive oil, helps people living in the Mediterranean region to maintain lower levels of cholesterol in blood, with a consequent lower risk for heart attacks and strokes.

CHOLESTEROL

Cholesterol is a fat-soluble steroid in blood that scientists think increases heart attacks and strokes by forming plaques and clogging blood vessels. Avoid cholesterol in foods even though the body makes most of the cholesterol in blood.

It seems best that people take in no more than 300 mg cholesterol per day; hard to do, since one chicken egg yolk contains 274 mg. Prescription drugs seem to provide an effective way to reduce cholesterol in blood.

SODIUM

The rule of thumb for salt intake (sodium chloride), set by different nutritional and medical organizations, suggests less than 2,000 to 5,000 mg per day. Medical scientists believe high salt intake can lead to high blood pressure, and this can lead to heart attacks and strokes. It seems best to rely on the natural amount of salt in foods and not add salt to food.

POTASSIUM

It seems unlikely that a potassium deficiency can occur. Still, various organizations recommend a minimum of 2,000 to 5,600 mg of potassium per day.

TOTAL CARBOHYDRATES

Carbohydrates provide some of the calories you need, as well as other chemical functions. Determine your need for them from the daily weight feedback trend.

FIBER

The rule of thumb for fiber (required for gastrointestinal health and for lowering cholesterol in blood) approaches 30 to 45 g per day. African natives take in more than 100 g per day. Go figure.

SUGARS

Avoid sugar (candy, cake, dessert, ice cream, junk foods, etc.), often called 'empty calories,' because these foods lack other nutrients, and because they augment tooth decay.

PROTEIN

We can only guess the daily requirement for protein, since it varies, as do the other nutrients, with age, weight, height, sex, activity, etc.

Fortunately, a rule of thumb works well enough. If you are a moderately active person, divide your weight in pounds by 2. This provides the minimum grams (g) of protein you require each day. If you are an active athlete, your weight in pounds can equal the grams of protein you need each day.

VITAMINS, MINERALS, & ANTIOXIDANTS

These substances overwhelm me because I find it tedious to calculate how much I get from each food, and how much of each I need per day. I avoid the entire confused state of affairs by taking one inexpensive capsule each day for vitamins & minerals, and one for antioxidants. Much easier and less expensive than you require, depending on the usual time-consuming hit-and-miss ways. I still eat salads, vegetables, and fruits, but with a more relaxed approach.

Some nutritionists say that if you eat a balanced diet, you do not have to take vitamin or mineral supplements." Here's the fallacy. How do you know if you eat a balanced diet? And even if you think so, how do you know you take in the required amounts of all the nutrients? I say take to inexpensive supplements for comfort.

WATER

The amount of water you require varies with body size, weather, activity, etc. Still, the rule of thumb advocates 4 to 8 glasses of water each day.

Other fluids, like milk, coffee, tea, and soup, do NOT substitute for water. Water flushes soluble wastes from the body, and these other fluids bring enough potential soluble wastes with them to cancel their watery function.

EATING RIGHT FOR LONGEVITY

Some people think or hope that special approaches to eating will enable them to live longer. More power to them.

It would seem more likely that some food will increase the quality of life by reducing stress and disease, thereby producing improved health.

In this regard, see the Sept/Oct 2009 issue of the AARP Bulletin (pages 22-24). It seems that on the 99-square mile Mediterranean Island of Ikaria, people tend to live longer and enjoy a better quality of life than in the USA.

For example, one in three Ikarians reaches 90, while only one in nine USA 'baby boomers' will. Also, Ikarians have 20% fewer cancer cases, 50% less heart disease, and about 10% less diabetes cases than Americans. Furthermore, Ikarians have no Alzheimer's disease or dementia, while 40% of Americans over 90 have these conditions.

The author of this study, Dan Buettner, listed 13 factors he thought might contribute to the health and longevity of these island people, of which 8 were foods. Buettner also wrote: "The Blue Zones: Lessons for Living Longer from the People Who Have Lived the Longest" in the 2008 volume of National Geographic. Worth looking into.

DO YOU KNOW HOW MUCH OF THESE NUTRIENTS (the Daily Value) YOU REQUIRE EACH DAY?

Calories?

Sodium?

Fiber?

Fat?

Potassium?

Protein?

Cholesterol?

Carbohydrate?

Vitamins?

Minerals?

ACTIVITY TABLE #4.

List Your Daily Required Amount of Each Nutrient (the Daily Values).

Calories:	cal
Calories from fat:	cal
Total fat:	g (grams)
Saturated fat:	g
Trans fat:	g
Polyunsaturated fat:	g
Monosaturated fat:	g
Cholesterol:	mg
Sodium:	mg
Potassium:	mg
Total carbohydrate:	g
Dietary fiber:	g
Soluble fiber:	g
Sugars:	g
Other carbohydrates:	g
Protein:	g
Vitamins:	% Daily Values (% DV)
Minerals:	% Daily Values (% DV)

ACTIVITY TABLE #5.

Determine Whether the Nutrients in the Foods You Listed in Activity Table #1 Meet Your Daily Required Amounts By Comparing It With Activity Table #4.

Which nutrients were low?

Which nutrients were high?

Which nutrients were just right?

What changes would you like to make in your food?

Comments:

ACTIVITY TABLE #6.

Devise an ideal full-day menu plan that will provide you with the required amounts of all the nutrients you need.

Breakfast:

Lunch:

Dinner:

Snacks:

What else:

Comments:

WARNING, BEFORE YOU DIET...

- Before dieting to lose weight, and before you start working out, **consult a Physician** to make sure you can do both safely.

- **Work out** when dieting to lose weight so you maintain your muscle mass.

- In addition, eat enough protein to insure your body does not break down your tissues, like your heart, kidneys, glands, muscles, and liver, to supply your brain and the nervous system with glucose for chemical energy, and amino acids for protein.

GOOD-MOOD FOODS & A HIGH-PROTEIN BREAKFAST

If you don't believe food affects your mood, try this. Skip several meals and you will feel hungry, and irritable, short tempered, perhaps sluggish and sleepy. Then eat something splendid and watch your mood and all those negative feelings reverse.

Scientific research and experimentation on myself suggest the following to me (see Appendix 1):

- A high protein breakfast (more than 25 g) tends to help people feel alert for up to 4 hours.

- A high fat breakfast tends to leave people feeling stuffed, sleepy, and irritable.

- A high carbohydrate breakfast tends to leave people feeling alert for about 2 hours, and sleepy and irritable after that.

In other words, a high protein meal tends to leave people (and me) feeling better, less irritable, and more alert than does a high fat or high carbohydrate meal. The effect seems to depend on the amount of insulin released from the pancreas gland, and on the ability of insulin to lower blood glucose.

Another take-home lesson: Make breakfast the biggest meal of the day, while cutting down on dinner. This tends to result in people feeling better with a greater sense of well-being. See also: "Food and Mood" by E. Somer, 1995; published by Henry Holt & Co; 460 pages.

WANTED: AN EASIER WAY TO PLAN

Determining the amount of nutrients in the food I eat, comparing the nutrients in what I eat to an ideal menu, judging the adequacy of my food intake on a daily basis, preparing food menus daily, making sure I get the nutrients I need and not losing muscle mass when I diet, makes for tedious & frustrating work, indeed.

No wonder people give up and either chuck it all, or cut corners on essential details to the detriment of the entire approach. We need an easier way to avoid this nightmare.

Because of this, I developed my simpler personal approach to eating right.

IV. WORKING OUT RIGHT: Strengthen & Tone Your Muscles, Improve Your Posture, Feel Fit

MY STORY

I worked out with weights and machines for about 40 years. This includes swimming (3 years ago 1 swam one mile) and cardiovascular training on a treadmill or cross trainer.

For the past 8 years, I worked out with a personal trainer two afternoons a week. I worked out alone a third afternoon a week, In addition, I currently do cardiovascular training on the treadmill for about an hour each time I go to the Fitness Center.

Work with my trainer enabled me to focus on good form. I was able to work out for less time, with less pain, and achieve overall better results.

The outcome of working out amazes and astonishes me. I have increased stamina; better muscle tone; more muscle mass; stronger legs, abs, upper body, lower back; better posture, a sense of well being; and I breathe easier as I walk up and down stairs and rush around.

WHY WORK OUT RIGHT?

Working out right provides many, many benefits: look good & feel fit, increased muscular stamina & endurance, joint & bone health (increase bone density & prevent osteoporosis), weight control (along with a sensible diet), heart health, increased energy, well-being, toned & strengthened muscles.

WORK OUT RIGHT WITH A TRAINER

You will experience many benefits if you work out with a trainer: better form, fewer accidents, less pain, better results, and more exact knowledge. If money presents a problem (and when doesn't it), hire a trainer to work with a group of people and share the cost between you.

Or work out with a friend (or a stranger who will become your friend), who has trained far longer than you, so you benefit from his or her experience and knowledge.

Before I worked out with a trainer, I worked out with experienced people (Dave and Sam) who generously gave me the benefit of their extensive knowledge. Then my trainer, Randy Ballard, focused me on form and commitment, and I learned determination, patience, and discipline.

FOCUS ON YOUR FORM

If you use correct form, you will avoid muscle strain that leads to pain and injuries. This means using a weight that allows you to carry out movements comfortably without the incredible straining that we sometimes observe in others. Easy does it: 'No Pain, All Gain' makes a splendid motto.

Learn form from a trainer or an experienced friend. Do not try to get it on your own unless you learn easily from thin air or books.

SCHEDULE YOUR WORKOUT RIGHT

The following schedule allows me enough time to workout right:

• 30 to 60 minutes: Warmup & cardiovascular workout.
• 30 to 45 minutes: Weight resistance workout with my trainer.
• 10 to 15 minutes: Cool down & stretching.
• 10 to 15 minutes: Hot tub & shower.

GIVE YOURSELF 'TOUGH LOVE'

We all find it hard to work out. We all know dozens of reasons to justify NOT working out. You know which ones you use, including the unconscious reasons you unawarely use.

Please stop doing this and treat yourself to 'tough love' to get you into a gym, spa, or fitness center. Arrange a feasible schedule so you can get there 2 to 3 times a week with enough time to work out and still do cardiovascular training. And keep getting help and advice from a trainer or an experienced friend. See these awesome books:

• 'Weight Training For Beginners' by Tony Gallagher (2003); published by Harper Resource, 96 pages. Outstanding book.

• 'The Complete Idiot's Guide to Weight Training' by Deidre Johnson-Cane, Jonathan Cane, and Joe Glickman (2005) Published by the Penguin Group, 304 pages. Nice book.

YOU WON'T LOSE MUCH WEIGHT WORKING OUT

A popular myth, 'work out and you will lose weight,' permeates the world of gyms, spas, and fitness centers. True, you do use up some calories during a workout session, but hardly enough.

You need to burn 3,500 calories to lose one pound of fat. To lose a pound of body weight a week, you need to use up 500 more calories per day, or to take in 500 calories less per day, than you require to maintain your body weight. In a workout session that lasts about one hour, you may use up about 200 to 350 calories. Only active athletes tend to burn up lots of calories, so they need to eat lots of calories or they will lose weight.

So how can you lose weight effectively and safely? You eat right to lose weight and work out to maintain muscle tone. Otherwise, you will lose protein (muscle) along with the fat. You also eat extra protein so your body doesn't break down your tissues, such as your heart, lungs, muscles, liver, kidney, glands, to obtain glucose (for chemical energy) and amino acids (for protein) for your brain.

You will not lose weight by working out unless you work out strenuously for 5 to 6 hours a day. Best to eat right instead.

WARM UP TO PREVENT INJURY

A decent warmup makes for a productive workout. Five to ten minutes of cardiovascular activity (on the treadmill or the cross trainer) will accomplish it. Ignore this at your peril. A good warmup can prevent sore muscles, injury, sprains, tendinitis, muscle or joint pain, etc.

DEHYDRATION

Sip water during your workout. You will feel better and prevent dehydration.

COOL DOWN AND STRETCH WHEN FINISHED

End your work out session with 3 to 4 minutes of slow walking, followed by 2 to 5 minutes of stretching. According to Randy Ballard, the head trainer at the First Health Fitness Center in Pinehurst, North Carolina, stretching reduces injuries, relaxes your muscles, and adds to the flexibility of your joints.

This results in easier workouts, enhances posture, and lowers muscle soreness. He recommends stretching until you feel tension, not pain, and holding the stretch for 15 to 30 seconds. Repeat one to two times, resting 10 to 15 seconds between each effort.

SCHEDULE TO START EATING & WORKING OUT RIGHT

The following schedule may help start you eating & working out right so you can lose & control your weight.

First week

- Obtain a physician's okay.
- Procure and start taking complete vitamins & minerals tablet once a day.
- Select a trainer and start working out three times a week.
- Start weighing yourself every other day at the same time of day. Important.
- Cut down on alcohol intake. Alcohol can lower discipline and motivation.

Second Week

- Fill out the six Activity Tables in this book.
- Start eating right.
- Cut food portions in half.
- No more intake of excess salt, fat, sugar.
- No desserts, fatty fried food, salty foods.
- Focus on foods that fill you up with a minimum of calories.

Third Week

- Start using Nutrition Facts labels to increase nutrients that promote health and
    decrease nutrients that do not promote health.
- Start high protein breakfasts and lunches.

Fourth Week

Copy my personal basic daily menu plan or devise one of your own, one that you repeat each day as I did, and thus reduce the tedium and frustration of food planning.

Your personal plan should deliver the daily nutrients you require with a minimum number of calories, so you can enjoy delicious balanced snacks that provide the additional calories you need. Determine the quantity of snacks you eat using the feedback from your every-other-day weighing. These weighings provide essential feedback.

Include ideas about what you will eat in restaurants, on road trips, and at dinner parties in your personal plan.

V. APPENDICES

Appendix I. Eating for Daily Alertness

STAY ALERT IN THE MORNING:
AVOID THE MIDMORNING SLUMP (the morning blahs)

The cause of the midmorning slump differs in different people. Research has indicated that a low-calorie, low-protein breakfast, <u>or</u> a high-carbohydrate breakfast causes it. You need to experiment with different breakfasts to find out what helps you.

A high carbohydrate breakfast produces short-lived alertness as the food raises the glucose level in your blood. This increase in glucose triggers an insulin flood into the bloodstream causing glucose levels to fall precipitously, and your alertness drops.

About an hour to two after you eat a high carbohydrate breakfast, your blood glucose drops so low that you probably feel irritable, and your midmorning slump sets in. To counteract this slump, many people take a break, drink a cup of coffee, and eat a "Danish" or a candy bar.

This starts the up-and-down alertness cycle again. Thus, most mornings start with you feeling good, followed by a "crash" in blood glucose levels, with a consequent decrease in your alertness and work effectiveness.

Evidence also exists that a high fat breakfast can also cause a midmorning slump.

RECOMMENDATION: Experiment with a high-protein breakfast containing at least 25 to 30 grams of protein to see if this helps your alertness and decreases your midmorning slump. The following Table provides sources of protein for your breakfast:

Sources of Protein for Breakfast:	
	<u>grams protein</u>
1 glass milk (skim milk) or low-calorie yogurt	8
2 eggs	12
4 tablespoons (2 ounces) low-fat cottage cheese	7
1 tablespoon (1 ounce) tuna fish	7
1 chicken thigh (remove skin before cooking)	15
3 oz steak (lean)	15-20
1 oz protein powder (100 % whey)	15
I/2 cup soybeans	10
2 tablespoons (1 ounce) wheat germ	9

Other high-protein foods include fish, shrimp, lamb, etc.

Sounds like too much effort? Not convinced? Almost everyone I know, including myself, who has tried a high-protein breakfast reports greater alertness and increased work effectiveness. The midmorning slump and the hunger for a "Danish" or a candy bar disappears. Try it and see.

AVOID THE AFTERNOON DOZE:
STAY ALERT AND PREVENT DROWSINESS AFTER LUNCH

The cause of drowsiness after lunch differs between people and at different times in the same person. Experiment with different foods to find out what affects you. People report the following foods as the most frequent causes of lower alertness after lunch (the afternoon doze):

- Too much fat (butter, hamburger, meat, gravy, salad dressing, etc.).

- Too much sugar (desserts, cakes, ice cream, cookies, candy, etc.).

- Not enough protein.

- Not enough, or too many, calories.

To help you find out what produces your mid-afternoon drowsiness, the following approach can prove useful:

- For lunch, eat a large salad with no dressing (dressing has 100 calories per tablespoon due to the fat in the oil), or with a small amount of low-cal dressing.

- Also drink a glass of skim milk (8-10 g protein with no fat).

- You may also eat a hard boiled egg (5-6 g protein).
- If you are still hungry, eat some fruit, such as an apple or a pear.
- Afternoon Snacks: Later in the afternoon, if you are hungry, drink a glass of skim milk and eat fruit (apple, pear, etc.).

If eating these foods helped you avoid drowsiness during the afternoon, you may discover the cause of your drowsiness by adding back your regular lunch foods, one at a time. Then if you feel drowsy, you will know the cause.

Sound like too much effort? The potential result, feeling alert in the afternoon, certainly makes it worth it. Besides, you do not have to experiment. Most people report that a lunch of a salad (with little or no dressing), skim milk, and a piece of fruit together with a mid-afternoon snack of skim milk and an apple or a pear does not cause drowsiness, and increases work effectiveness.

My regular lunch, consisting of milk whey Protein Powder, Fiber One cereal, and skim milk, does not lower alertness.

SOME SCIENTIFIC REFERENCES

Thorn, G.W., J.T. Quinby and M. Clinton (1943). A comparison of the metabolic effects of isocaloric meals of varying compositions with special reference to the prevention of postprandial hypoglycemic symptoms. Annals of Internal Medicine 18:913-919.

Orent-Keiles, E. and L.F. Hallman (1949). The breakfast meal in relation to blood sugar values. U.S. Department of Agriculture Circular 827.

Spring, B.,0. Maller, J. Wurtman, L. Digman, and L. Cozolino (1985). Effects of protein and carbohydrate meals on mood and performance: Interactions with sex and age. Journal Psychiatric Research 17:155-157.

See also: "Food and Mood" by E. Somer (1995); published by Henry Holt & Co; 460 pages.

APPENDIX II. Feeling Full*

When dieting to lose weight, you need to eat foods that fill you up and satisfy your hunger with a minimum intake of calories. Research has shown these foods tend to have greater amounts of water, fiber, and/or protein (like vegetables, fruits, lean meats).

On the other hand, foods composed mainly of carbohydrates and/or fat, do not satisfy your hunger until you eat many more calories of them, thus undermining your attempt to lose weight.

SOME FOODS THAT SATISFY YOU WITH FEWER INTAKE OF CALORIES

(These foods have higher amounts of water, fiber, and/or protein)

Bean sprouts

Watermelon

Grapefruit

Carrots

Oranges

Fish, broiled

Chicken breast

Apples

Sirloin steak

Oatmeal

Popcorn

SOME FOODS THAT SATISFY YOU BUT NEED EXTRA CALORIES TO DO IT

(These foods have high amounts of carbohydrates and/or fat)

Baked potato

Low-fat yogurt

Banana

Macaroni and cheese

Brown rice

Spaghetti

White rice

Pizza

Peanuts

Ice cream

White bread

Raisins

Snickers Bar

Honey

Sugar (sucrose)

Glucose

Potato chips

Butter

Factor this in when attempting to diet to lose weight.

*Adapted from nutritiondata.com (Fullness Factor)

MATZOS CRACKERS

Manischewitz's matzos cracker, made with whole wheat flour and water, provides an excellent filling food with a low number of calories.

The Nutritional Facts label indicates that 12 matzos crackers weigh one ounce and contain 110 calories with no calories from fat; they also contains no cholesterol or sodium, 40 mg potassium, 25 g carbohydrate, and 3 g protein. Great for snacks.

Appendix III. 1984 HANDOUT TO MY NUTRITION CLASS

PRUDENT, SENSIBLE, AND EFFECTIVE FOOD HABITS

Prepared by Edward Glassman, Ph.D.

I based this 1984 handout for my nutrition class on a variety of sources:

- U.S. Dietary Goals of the Select Committee on Nutrition and Human Needs, U.S. Senate, December 1977
- The Prudent Diet of the American Heart Association
- The Recommended Dietary Allowances of the Food and Nutrition Board of the National Research Council of the National Academy of Sciences (U.S.)

SUGGESTION	REASON
1. BALANCED FOOD INTAKE There are nutrients about which we know little concerning the amount required and in which foods they exist. In addition, there may be undiscovered nutrients. Eat in a balanced way to insure intake of these nutrients. For a balanced food intake, eat a variety of foods including meat, vegetables, fruit, starch, fat, and milk.	1. There are nutrients about which we know very little concerning the amount required and in which foods they exist. In addition, there may be undiscovered nutrients. Eat in a balanced way to insure intake of these nutrients.

SUGGESTION	REASON

2. HIGH PROTEIN BREAKFAST

Eat a breakfast containing at least 20-25 g of protein.

2. The research of Thorn et al. (1943) and Orent-Keiles and Hallman (1949) suggests that a high protein breakfast delays the onset of fatigue and restlessness due to the fall of blood glucose levels that follow a high carbohydrate or a high fat breakfast.

3. SALT

Limit intake of sodium (salt) to less than 5 g per day. To do this, salt your food sparingly or not at all; the natural salt content of food is enough. Be aware that canned and other processed foods contain high amounts of salt.

3. High salt intake is thought to put an unnecessary stress on the kidneys and may lead to or increase hypertension (high blood pressure). Hypertension has been shown to lead to heart disease and stroke.

4. SUGAR

Greatly reduce or eliminate sugar in your diet. This includes candy, cake, ice cream, honey, most desserts, soft drinks, sweetened cereals, brown sugar, table sugar, molasses. Be aware that food labeled as containing sucrose, dextrose, dextrin, honey, brown sugar, glucose, cane syrup, molasses, corn syrup, etc., contain sugar.

4. Sugar causes harm in at least 3 ways: First, research clearly shows that sugar is one of the major causes of dental caries and gingivitis by enabling the bacteria in dental plaque to form harmful organic acids and toxic chemicals. Second, sugar suppresses your appetite so you will not take in the nutrients you need. Third, ingesting sugar may lead to low blood glucose levels causing fatigue and irritability an hour or so after ingestion.

SUGGESTION	REASON

5. OVERWEIGHT

Change your food habits if you are overweight. Increase consumption of fruits, vegetables, salads, whole grains, nonfat milk, fish. Eliminate or reduce butter, cream, margarine, fatty meats, deserts, sugar, oil, nuts, fats, etc

5. Research indicates that overweight leads to or aggravates heart disease, hypertension, diabetes, stroke, etc. Over-consumption of food represents a major nutritional hazard in the American population today

6. SATURATED FAT

Reduce intake of saturated fats by cutting down on beef, pork, sheep, whole milk, cream, coconut oil. Partially replace saturated fats with polyunsaturated fats found in safflower oil, corn oil, and other oils that remain liquid in refrigerator. Increase the ratio of Polyunsaturated fatty acids to Saturated
Fatty acids (the P/S RATIO) in your diet so it exceeds 'one.'

6. Research suggests that a higher P/S ratio of fatty acids leads to lower levels and a higher HDL (good cholesterol) / LDL (bad cholesterol) ratio in the blood. This can result in lower heart disease and stroke. This is thought more effective than lowering cholesterol in the diet, although both approaches make sense.

7. POLYUNSATURATED FAT

Reduce intake of polyunsaturated fat (also see 6 above)

7. Research associates a high intake of polyunsaturated fat with increased incidence of colon cancer.

SUGGESTION	REASON

8. CHOLESTEROL

Reduce intake of foods that contain cholesterol. This includes butter, beef, lamb, pork, mutton, eggs. Substitute fish, skinned chicken, turkey, etc., not cooked in fat.

8. Research shows that high levels of blood cholesterol increase the risk of heart disease and stroke. Lowering cholesterol levels in the food you eat can lower blood cholesterol.

9. STARCHY FOODS

Obtain calories mostly from starchy foods like bread, potatoes, whole grains, etc.
fatty acids (the P/S ratio) in your diet to 'one' or better.

9. Sugar and fats, also a source of calories, have harmful side effects (see 4,5,6,7 above).

10. FIBER:

Increase intake of foods that contain fiber. These include bran, whole grains, celery, carrots, salads.

10. Normal digestive functions and movement through the gut is thought to be helped by the presence of fiber.

11. SYSTEMATIC APPROACH:

Use the R.D.A. and the Food Exchange List as guide to preparing daily menu plans.

11. It is extremely difficult to maintain nutrient adequacy and balance without a systematic daily approach.

SUGGESTION	REASON
12. FAST FOOD RESTAURANTS: Avoid eating too often in fast food restaurants	12. Although food served in these places is not always junk food, research has shown that the number of calories is very high due to high amounts of carbohydrate and fat. According to Young et al. (1979) and Consumer Reports (1979), the average meal at a fast food place can provide one-half to two-thirds the calories needed daily by an adult. In addition, fast food contains high amounts of salt (see 3 above). Too many calories, fat, carbohydrate, and salt.
13. CALCIUM Insure adequate R.D.A. intake of calcium by drinking one quart of skim milk per day, or a food high in calcium.	13. Research indicates that many individuals do not have adequate intake of calcium. This deficiency is thought to lead to osteoporosis, a softening of bone, in later life. Osteoporosis is especially prevalent in women after menopause.
14. IRON Insure adequate intake of iron, by supplement if necessary.	14. Research indicates that most individuals, especially women, do not take in adequate iron. Analysis of typical American diets confirm this.

SUGGESTION	REASON

15. CHILDREN'S FOOD HABITS

Expose your infants and children to the foods you want them to eat later in life. Oo not expose them to foods that are high in sugar, fats and salt.

15. Infancy and childhood is when we learn most of our food habits. Do not . expose your children to foods you know to be harmfull. Do not eat these foods yourself

.

16. CRASH DIETS

Avoid crash diets with very low caloric intakes.

16. Crash diets are inadequate and even hazardous. They are low in salt and the large initial weight loss is due to loss of water. This is gained back just as fast when you resume your regular eating habits. Such low caloric intake leads to a breakdown of muscle protein to generate glucose for brain energy. Glucose comes either from the food you eat or from the breakdown of protein in muscle and other tissues. Fat cannot be used for this purpose.

17. SNACKS

Eat an apple (or other fruit) and drink a glass of skim milk instead of sugary non-protein snacks.

17. Research shows that the best snack is a glass of milk (8 to 10 g protein) and a fruit (carbohydrate plus bulk).

.

You may want to consider reducing the following in your food

HIGH SUGAR

Any commercial product labeled with sugar, dextrose can syrup, dextrin, molasses, brown sugar, corn syrup, sucrose, glucose, honey, etc.

HIGH SATURATED FAT

Any commercial product containing hydrogenated oil of any type.
All fat fried foods,
Dairy cream

HIGH SALT

Almost all canned and processed foods such as vegetables, soups, meats, fish, chili, stuffing mixes, pickled vegetables, vegetable juices, unless labeled otherwise.

For example:

Presweetened cereals
Commercial granola
Sweetened canned and frozen juices
Candy
Cakes
Most deserts
Ice cream
Milk shakes
Honey
Molasses
Brown sugar
Jam, jelly
Syrup

For example:

Pastries, donuts, cakes
Fried potatoes
Fried chicken
Potato chips
Corn chips
Cream cheese and most other cheeses
Sour cream
Whole milk
Butter, most margarine
Beef or veal
Lamb or mutton
Pork, ham or bacon
Canned meats Peanuts
Duck, goose

For example:

Buttermilk
Ham
Bacon
Corned beef
Pastrami
Sausage
Frankfurters
Wurst
Salami
Smoked meat and fish
Salted meat and fish
Canned and processed food
Processed cheese

PLEASE WRITE YOUR NUTRITION GOALS FOR EACH OF THE FOLLOWING:

1. Balanced Food Intake:

2. High Protein Breakfast:

3. Salt:

4. Sugar:

5. Overweight:

6. Saturated Fat:

7. Polyunsaturated Fat:

8. Cholesterol:

9. Starchy Foods:

10. Fiber:

11. Systematic Approach:

12. Fast Food Restaurants:

13. Calcium:

14. Iron:

15. Your Children's Food Habits:

16. Crash Diets:

17. Snacks:

USE THE 'NUTRITION FACTS' LABEL TO EAT HEALTHIER*

* (Adapted from the US Food and Drug Administration)

The Nutrition Facts label helps people determine what NUTRIENTS exist in the food they eat. Comparing these labels will help you know which foods have lower fat or fewer calories, which foods make healthy snacks, and which used for special diets.

SERVING SIZE

Check the serving size and number of servings in the package. The Nutrition Facts Label bases information on ONE serving, but many packages contain more than one. If you unknowingly double the servings you eat, you double your intake of calories and nutrients. If the label states that one serving equals 3 pieces and 100 calories, and you eat 6 pieces, you've eaten 2 servings, and twice the number of calories and fat. Check to see if the serving size varies between brands.

CALORIES

The Nutrition Facts label indicates the number of calories per serving and the calories from fat in each serving. Fat-free doesn't mean calorie-free. Items with less fat may have as many calories as full-fat versions.

FIBER, VITAMINS A & C, POTASSIUM, CALCIUM, AND IRON

Use the Nutrition Facts label to increase nutrients that promote good health and protect you from disease. Some people don't get enough fiber, vitamins A and C, potassium, calcium, and iron, so choose the brands with the higher levels for these nutrients.

DAILY VALUE (DV) & % DAILY VALUE (%DV)

The Daily Value (DV) equals the amount of that particular nutrient you require each day (see Activity Table #4).

The % Daily Value (% DV) tells you what percent of your total daily requirement one serving of that food supplies you, and indicates how much a specified amount of that food contributes to your daily diet. In other words, the % DV enables you to know how much of that required nutrient is in one serving of that food.

The % DV helps you determine if a food contains high or low amounts of a nutrient: note that 5% DV or less represents a low amount and 20% DV or more represents a high amount.

Usually the Nutrition Facts label bases the % DV on a 2,000-calorie diet. Even though you may not take in that number of calories per day, the % DV still provides useful information about a nutrient.

FAT

Different types of fat affect your health. To reduce your risk of heart disease, use the Nutrition Facts label to select foods that are lowest in saturated fat, Trans fat, and cholesterol. Trans fat doesn't have a % DV, but consume very little because it increases your risk of heart disease.

CHOLESTEROL

To lower blood cholesterol, replace saturated and trans fats with monounsaturated and polyunsaturated fats found in fish, nuts, olives, and vegetable oils.

SODIUM

Use the Nutritional Facts label to limit sodium and help reduce your risk of high blood pressure and consequent heart disease & stroke.

FIBER

Fiber and sugars are types of carbohydrates. Sources of fiber, like fruits, vegetables, beans, and whole grains, can reduce your risk of heart disease and improve digestive functioning. Use the Nutrition Facts labels to choose foods high in fiber.

GRAINS

You can't always identify whole grain foods by color or name, such as multigrain or wheat. Look for the "whole" grain listed first in the Ingredients list on the bottom of the Nutrition Facts label, such as whole wheat, brown rice, or whole oats.

SUGAR

There isn't a % DV for sugar, but you can compare the sugar content in grams among products. Use the Nutrition Facts label to limit foods with added sugars (sucrose, glucose, fructose, corn or maple syrup). These add empty calories but not other nutrients (junk foods). Avoid foods with added sugars as one of the first few items in the Ingredients list at the bottom of the Nutrition Facts label.

PROTEIN

Most people get plenty of protein, but not always from the healthiest, low fat, sources. When choosing a food for its protein content, choose lean, low-fat, or fat free sources, such as meat, poultry, dry beans, milk and milk products.

*Adapted from the US Food and Drug Administration

SAMPLE 'NUTRITION FACTS' LABEL*

Nutrition Facts

Serving Size 1 cup (228g)
Servings Per Container 2

Amount Per Serving

Calories 260 Calories from fat 120

% Daily Value*

Total Fat 13g	**20%**
Saturated Fat 5g	**25%**
Cholesterol 30mg	**10%**
Sodium 660mg	**28%**
Total Carbohydrate 31g	**10%**
Dietary Fiber 0g	**0%**
Sugars 5g	
Protein 5g	

Vitamin A 4%	●	Vitamin C 2%	
Calcium 15%	●	Iron 4%	

* Percent Daily Values are based on a 2,000 calorie diet. Your daily value may be higher or lower depending on your calorie needs:

		Calories:	2,000	2,500
Total Fat	Less than		65g	80g
Sat Fat	Less than		20g	25g
Cholesterol	Less than		300mg	300mg
Sodium	Less than		2,400mg	2,400mg
Total Carbohydrate			300g	375g
Dietary Fiber			25g	30g

Calories per gram:
Fat 9 * Carbohydrate 4 * Protein 4

*TAKEN FROM THE USDA

HOW TO UNDERSTAND AND USE THE NUTRITION FACTS LABEL

(The Following is Adapted from the US FDA)

CONTENTS

- The Nutrition Facts Panel - An Overview

- The Serving Size

- Calories (and Calories from Fat)

- The Nutrients: How Much?

- Understanding the Footnote

- How the Daily Values (DV) Relate to the %DVs

- The Percent Daily Value (%DV)

- Quick Guide to %DV

- Nutrients With a %DV but No Weight Listed - Spotlight on Calcium

- Nutrients Without a %DV: Trans Fats, Protein, and Sugars

THE NUTRITION FACTS LABEL

The information in the top section of the Nutrition Facts label varies with each food product and contains product-specific information (serving size, calories, and nutrient information).

The bottom section contains a footnote with the required daily amount for each nutrient. These are listed as the Daily Values (DVs) for 2,000 and 2,500 calorie diets. The % DV provides recommended dietary requirements for important nutrients, including fats, sodium and fiber.

NUTRITIONAL FACTS LABEL FOR MACARONI & CHEESE

Nutrition Facts

Serving Size 1 cup (228g)
Servings Per Container 2

Total Fat 12g	18%
Saturated Fat 3g	15%
Trans Fat 3g	
Cholesterol 30mg	10%
Sodium 470mg	20%
Total Carbohydrate 31g	10%
Dietary Fiber 0g	0%
Sugars 5g	
Protein 5g	
Vitamin A	4%
Vitamin C	2%
Calcium	20%
Iron	4%

	Calories:	2,000	2,500
* Percent Daily Values are based on a 2,000 calorie diet. Your Daily Values may be higher or lower depending on your calorie needs.			
Total Fat	Less than	65g	80g
Sat Fat	Less than	20g	25g
Cholesterol	Less than	300mg	300mg
Sodium	Less than	2,400mg	2,400mg
Total Carbohydrate		300g	375g
Dietary Fiber		25g	30g

Serving Size

The size of the serving on the food package influences the number of calories and the nutrient amounts listed on the top part of the label. Pay attention to the serving size, and especially to how many servings there are in the food package.

Calories (and Calories from Fat)

Calories on the Nutritional Facts label provide a measure of how much energy you get from a serving of this food. Many Americans consume more calories than they need without meeting recommended daily intakes for a number of other nutrients. The calorie section of the label can help you manage your weight. The number of servings you eat determines the number of calories you take in.

Amount Per Serving	
Calories 250	Calories from Fat 110

In this Nutrition Facts label, there are 250 calories in one serving of this macaroni and cheese. How many calories from fat exist in ONE serving? Answer: 110 calories, which means almost half the calories in a single serving come from fat. If you ate the entire package, you would consume two servings, or 500 calories, and 220 calories would come from fat. Experts believe that eating too many calories per day can produce overweight and obesity.

The Nutrients: How Much?

Look at the top of the nutrient section in the sample label. It shows you some key nutrients that affect your health and separates them into two main groups: those which you want to limit intake & those which you want to exceed intake...

Limit Your Intake of These Nutrients

Total Fat 12g	**18%**
Saturated Fat 3g	**15%**
Trans Fat 3g	
Cholesterol 30mg	**10%**
Sodium 470mg	**20%**

The nutrients listed first on this Nutrition Facts label are the ones Americans generally eat in adequate amounts, and even too much. Limit these Nutrients. Eating too much fat, saturated fat, trans fat, cholesterol, or sodium may increase your risk of heart disease, stroke, some cancers, or high blood pressure. Important: Health experts recommend that you keep your intake of saturated fat, trans fat and cholesterol very low.

Get Enough of These Nutrients

Dietary Fiber 0g	0%
Vitamin A	4%
Vitamin C	2%
Calcium	20%
Iron	4%

Many people don't get enough dietary fiber, vitamin A, vitamin C, calcium, and iron in their diets. Eating enough of these nutrients can improve your health and help reduce the risk of some diseases and ailments.

For example, getting enough calcium may reduce the risk of osteoporosis, a condition that results in brittle bones as one ages (see calcium section below). Eating a diet high in dietary fiber promotes healthy bowel function.

Additionally, a diet rich in fruits, vegetables, and grain products that contain dietary fiber, particularly soluble fiber, and low in saturated fat and cholesterol may reduce your risk of heart disease.

You can use the Nutrition Facts label not only to help limit those nutrients you want to cut back on, but also to increase those nutrients you need to eat in greater amounts.

The Footnote on the Bottom of the Nutrition Facts Label

	Calories:	2,000	2,500
Total Fat	Less than	65g	80g
Sat Fat	Less than	20g	25g
Cholesterol	Less than	300mg	300mg
Sodium	Less than	2,400mg	2,400mg
Total Carbohydrate		300g	375g
Dietary Fiber		25g	30g

* Percent Daily Values are based on a 2,000 calorie diet. Your Daily Values may be higher or lower depending on your calorie needs.

Daily Value (DV) and % Daily Value (% DV)

The Daily Value (DV) represents the recommended amount of that nutrient that you require each day. The % Daily Value (% DV) represents the percent of the Daily Value you will take in if you eat one serving of this food. It will tell you if this food provides an effective source of the nutrient, since the higher the % DV, the better the source.

Note the * (asterisk) used after the heading "% Daily Value" on the Nutrition Facts label. It refers to the lower part of the nutrition label, which tells you that the "% DVs are based on a 2,000 or 2,500 calorie diet.

Look at the amounts circled. These are the amounts, the DV, you require daily of each nutrient, and are based on the advice of public health experts. The DVs are recommended daily amounts required for each nutrient based on a 2,000 or 2,500 calorie diet.

How the Daily Values Relate to the % DVs

Look at the Table below to see how the DVs relate to the % DVs and dietary guidance. For each nutrient listed, there exists a DV, a % DV, and dietary advice or a goal. If you follow this dietary advice, you will stay within public health experts' recommended upper or lower limits for the nutrients listed based on a 2,000 calorie daily diet.

DVs and % DVs Based on a 2,000 Calorie Diet

Nutrient (Required Daily Amount)	DV	% DV	Goal
Total Fat	65 g	= 100% DV	Eat Less Of
Saturated Fat	20 g	= 100% DV	Eat Less Of
Cholesterol	300 mg	= 100% DV	Eat Less Of
Sodium	2400 mg	= 100% DV	Eat Less Of
Total Carbohydrate	300 g	= 100% DV	Eat At least
Dietary Fiber	25 g	= 100% DV	Eat At least

Upper Limit: Eat "less" than this amount...

The nutrients that have upper daily limits are listed first on the footnote of larger Nutrition Facts labels, and on the Macaroni & Cheese example above. Upper limits means that you should eat less than the Daily Value per day. For example, the DV for Saturated fat equals 20 g. This amount equals the 100% DV for this nutrient, so eat less than 20 g or 100% of the DV each day.

Lower Limit - Eat "At least" this amount...

The DV for Dietary Fiber is 25 g, which equals the 100% DV. This means the experts recommend that you eat at least 25 g, and more, of dietary fiber per day,

The DV for Total Carbohydrate is 300 g or 100% DV. The experts recommend 300 g for a daily diet based on 2,000 calories, but can vary, depending on your daily intake of fat and protein.

The Percent Daily Value (% DV):

The % Daily Values (% DVs) are based on the Daily Value recommendations for key nutrients, but only for a 2,000 calorie daily diet, not 2,500 calories. You may not know how many calories you consume in a day, but you can still use the % DV as a frame of reference no matter how many calories you consume each day.

The % DV helps you determine if a serving of food is high or low in a particular nutrient. Note: a few nutrients, like trans fat and protein, do not have a % DV; they will be discussed later.

Quick Guide to % DV

5% DV or less represents a low amount, while 20% DV or more represents a high amount.

	% Daily Value*
Total Fat 12g	18%
Saturated Fat 3g	15%
Trans Fat 3g	
Cholesterol 30mg	10%
Sodium 470mg	20%
Total Carbohydrate 31g	10%
Dietary Fiber 0g	0%
Sugars 5g	
Protein 5g	
Vitamin A	4%
Vitamin C	2%
Calcium	20%
Iron	4%

Nutrients With a % DV but No Weight Listed: Calcium

Look at the % DV for calcium on food packages so you know how much one serving contributes to the total amount you need per day, the DV. Experts advise adults consume 1,000 mg or 100% DV in a daily 2,000 calorie diet. Note the Nutrition Facts label only lists a % DV for calcium, not an amount.

Experts advise that adolescents, especially girls, consume 1400 mg (130% DV) and post-menopausal women consume 1,200 mg (120% DV) of calcium daily. The DV for calcium on food labels is 1,000 mg.

Always check the label for calcium because you can't make assumptions about the amount of calcium in specific food categories. Example: the amount of calcium in milk, whether skim or whole, is generally the same per serving, whereas the amount of calcium in the same size yogurt container (8 oz) varies from 20 to 45% DV.

Nutrients Without a % DV: Trans Fats, Protein, and Sugars

Note that Trans fat, Sugars and Protein do not have a % DV on the Nutrition Facts label.

Trans Fat

Experts do not provide enough information for trans fat that FDA believes is sufficient to establish a Daily Value. Scientific reports associate trans fat and saturated fat with raising blood LDL (bad cholesterol) levels, so both increase your risk for coronary heart disease. Health experts recommend that you minimize your intake of saturated fat, trans fat, and cholesterol.

Protein

A % DV must be listed if a product makes a claim for protein, such as "high in protein." Otherwise, unless the food is meant for infants and children under 4 years old, no % DV is needed. Current scientific evidence indicates that people in the USA take in adequate protein, and thus protein intake does not comprise a public health concern for adults and children over 4 years of age.

Plain Yogurt		Fruit Yogurt	

Nutrition Facts		**Nutrition Facts**	
Serving Size 1 container (226g)		Serving Size 1 container (227g)	
Amount Per Serving		**Amount Per Serving**	
Calories 110 Calories from Fat 0		**Calories** 240 Calories from Fat 25	
	% Daily Value*		% Daily Value*
Total Fat 0g	0 %	**Total Fat** 3g	4 %
Saturated Fat 0g	0 %	Saturated Fat 1.5g	9 %
Trans Fat 0g		Trans Fat 0g	
Cholesterol Less than 5mg	1 %	**Cholesterol** 15mg	5 %
Sodium 160mg	7 %	**Sodium** 140mg	6 %
Total Carbohydrate 15g	5 %	**Total Carbohydrate** 46g	15 %
Dietary Fiber 0g	0 %	Dietary Fiber Less than 1g	3 %
Sugars 10g		Sugars 44g	
Protein 13g		**Protein** 9g	
Vitamin A 0 % • Vitamin C	4 %	Vitamin A 2 % • Vitamin C	4 %
Calcium 45 % • Iron	0 %	Calcium 35 % • Iron	0 %
*Percent Daily Values are based on a 2,000 calorie diet. Your Daily Values may be higher or lower depending on your calorie needs.		*Percent Daily Values are based on a 2,000 calorie diet. Your Daily Values may be higher or lower depending on your calorie needs.	

Sugars

No Daily Value has been established for sugars because no recommendations exist for the total amount to eat in a day. The sugars listed on the Nutrition Facts label include naturally occurring sugars (like those in fruit and milk) as well as those added to a food or drink. Always check the Ingredients list for added sugars.

Look at the Nutrition Facts labels for the two yogurt examples above. The plain yogurt has 10 g of sugars, the fruit yogurt has 44 g of sugars in one serving.

Now look at the Ingredient lists at the bottom of each label. Ingredients are listed in descending order of weight (from most to least). Note that no added sugars or sweeteners exist in the list of ingredients for the **plain** yogurt, even though 10 g of sugars are listed on the Nutrition Facts label. This is because there are no added sugars in plain yogurt, only the naturally occurring sugars (lactose in the milk).

The effect of added sugar on the calories of the two yogurts bogles the mind, from 110 calories in a container of plain yogurt to 240 calories in a container of the fruit yogurt. This difference can interfere if you want to lose weight.

Plain Yogurt - contains no added sugars and 110 calories.

INGREDIENTS: CULTURED PASTEURIZED GRADE A NONFAT MILK, WHEY PROTEIN CONCENTRATE, PECTIN, CARRAGEENAN.

Fruit Yogurt - contains added sugars and 240 calories.

INGREDIENTS: CULTURED GRADE A REDUCED FAT MILK, APPLES, HIGH FRUCTOSE CORN SYRUP, CINNAMON, NUTMEG, NATURAL FLAVORS, AND PECTIN. CONTAINS ACTIVE YOGURT AND L. ACIDOPHILUS CULTURES.

If you are concerned about your intake of sugars, make sure that the Ingredients list does not list added sugars as one of the first few ingredients. Other names for added sugars include: corn syrup, high-fructose corn syrup, fruit juice concentrate, maltose, dextrose, sucrose, honey, and maple syrup.

To limit nutrients that have no % DV, like trans fat and sugars, compare the Nutrition Facts labels of similar products and choose the food with the lowest amount.

MILK COMPARISONS: See the Nutrition Facts labels below for two kinds of milk, one for "Reduced Fat," the other for "Nonfat" milk. Each serving size equals one cup. Which has more calories and more saturated fat? Which one has more calcium?

| REDUCED FAT MILK | NONFAT MILK |
| 2% Fat | NO FAT |

# Nutrition Facts	# Nutrition Facts
Serving Size 1 cup (236ml) Servings Per Container 1	Serving Size 1 cup (236ml) Servings Per Container 1
Amount Per Serving	**Amount Per Serving**
Calories 120 Calories from Fat 45	**Calories** 80 Calories from Fat 0
% Daily Value*	% Daily Value*
Total Fat 5g **8%**	**Total Fat** 0g 0%
Saturated Fat 3g **15%**	Saturated Fat 0g 0%
Trans Fat 0g	*Trans* Fat 0g
Cholesterol 20mg 7%	**Cholesterol** Less than 5mg 0%
Sodium 120mg 5%	**Sodium** 120mg 5%
Total Carbohydrate 11g 4%	**Total Carbohydrate** 11g 4%
Dietary Fiber 0g 0%	Dietary Fiber 0g 0%
Sugars 11g	Sugars 11g
Protein 9g 17%	**Protein** 9g 17%
Vitamin A 10% • Vitamin C 4% Calcium 30% • Iron 0% • Vitamin D 25%	Vitamin A 10% • Vitamin C 4% Calcium 30% • Iron 0% • Vitamin D 25%
*Percent Daily Values are based on a 2,000 calorie diet. Your daily values may be higher or lower depending on your calorie needs.	*Percent Daily Values are based on a 2,000 calorie diet. Your daily values may be higher or lower depending on your calorie needs.

ANSWER: As you can see, they both have the same amount of calcium, but the nonfat milk has no saturated fat and has 40 calories less per serving than the reduced fat milk. In addition, nonfat milk has 100 calories less than whole fat (4%) milk. *(Adapted from the USDA: Dated June 2000, updated July 2003, and November 2004).

PROTEIN POWDER*

Milk & Egg

Serving Size 1 Scoop (35g) Servings Per Container 45

(3.5lb Container)

	Amount Per Serving	%DV
Calories	112	
Total Carbohydrate	4g	2%*
Sugars	4g	**
Total Fat	0g	0%
Protein	24g	48%*
Vitamin A (as beta carotene)	2500IU	50%
Vitamin C (as ascorbic acid)	30mg	50%
Vitamin D (as ergocalciferol)	200IU	50%
Thiamin (as mononitrate)	750mcg	50%
Riboflavin	850mcg	50%
Niacin (as niacinimide)	10mg	50%
Vitamin B6 (as pyridoxine HCl)	1mg	50%
Vitamin B12 (as cyanocobalamin)	3mcg	50%
Biotin	75mcg	25%
Calcium (as sulfate)	500mg	50%
Iron	180mcg	<2%
Magnesium (as oxide)	100mg	25%
Sodium	145mg	6%*
Protein Enzyme Complex	50mg	
Papain		**
Bromelain		**

Other Ingredients: Premium Protein Blend (consisting of calcium caseinate, lactalbumin and egg white albumin), dextrose, natural flavors, lecithin, papain, bromelain.

Recommended Use: Mix 1-2 level scoops in a blender with 12 oz. of your favorite beverage, or as directed. Intense training requires a daily intake of about 1g of protein per 2.2 pounds of body weight.

Milk & Egg Protein, a combination of milk protein (casein & lactalbumin), a Milk and egg protein (albumin), contains only slow-acting, easily digestible proteins, readily used by your body. To optimize your muscle gains and to prevent muscle breakdown, we recommend you take in protein every three hours.*Adapted from an advertisement for body builders**.

SOME SATISFIED READERS IN MY FAMILY

Hi Dad - I read your book last night. Great job.

It was very interesting and informative. I put wheat germ on my oatmeal this morning to get more protein at your suggestion! Thanks for the tip.

You should put more in it about fitness. I have found that even though you may not lose weight by working out, you do firm up your body and that makes you feel like you are losing weight. It also makes you feel so good. Quite an amazing benefit.
-----ELLEN

I like it, Dad! It's catchy!
Nick was reading your nutrition book today, and
he really took it to heart. He is going to start eating more
protein in the morning. You made an impact!
-----SUSAN

THE AUTHOR, EDWARD GLASSMAN, IN HIS 80TH YEAR

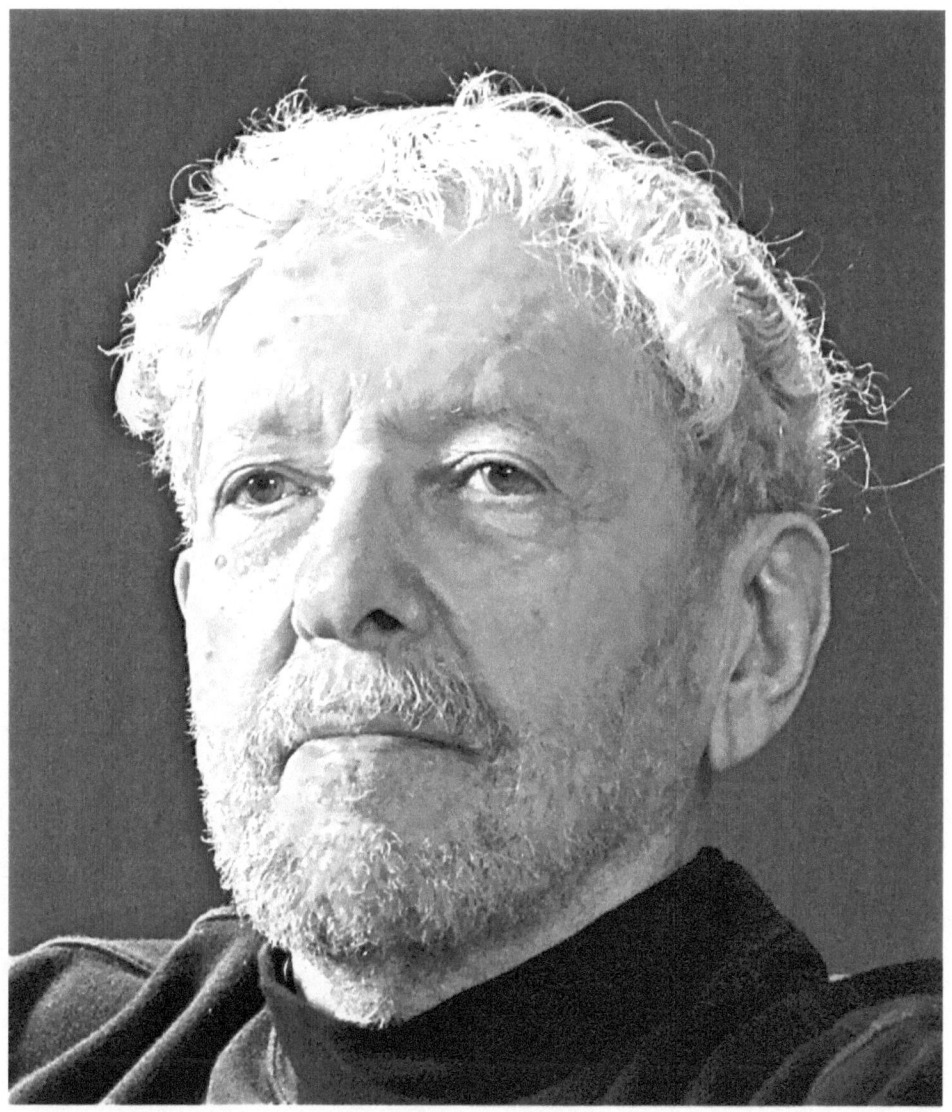

THE AUTHOR, EDWARD GLASSMAN, AT AGE ONE YEAR.

www.ingramcontent.com/pod-product-compliance
Lightning Source LLC
Chambersburg PA
CBHW050500290526
45786CB00006B/2365